T0065564

PREPARATION FOR THE END

MORAL AND NATURAL LAW

Claire Power Murphy

Editor: Deanie Humphrys-Dunne
Design: Phillip Haveard

authorHOUSE®

AuthorHouse™
1663 Liberty Drive
Bloomington, IN 47403
www.authorhouse.com
Phone: 1 (800) 839-8640

Published by AuthorHouse 08/09/2016

ISBN: 978-1-5246-2218-3 (sc)
ISBN: 978-1-5246-2217-6 (e)

Library of Congress Control Number: 2016912476

Print information available on the last page.

Disclaimer: Author Claire Power Murphy is not a Medical Doctor nor is her Foundation a Medical Facility. The Marvelous Healing Powers of Nature, shared as part of this book, are not to be taken as specific recommendations for any one person. Before undertaking any health activity, the services of a Medical Doctor or a Healthcare Professional are recommended.

This book is printed on acid-free paper.

Because of the dynamic nature of the Internet, any web addresses or links contained in this book may have changed since publication and may no longer be valid. The views expressed in this work are solely those of the author and do not necessarily reflect the views of the publisher, and the publisher hereby disclaims any responsibility for them.

Scripture quotations marked KJV are from the Holy Bible, King James Version (Authorized Version). First published in 1611. Quoted from the KJV Classic Reference Bible, Copyright © 1983 by The Zondervan Corporation.

TABLE
OF
CONTENTS

Claire Power Murphy

SECTIONS

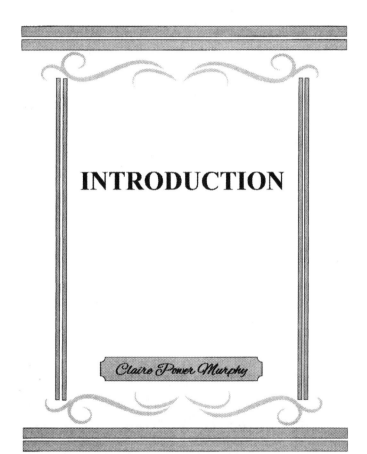

INTRODUCTION

Claire Power Murphy

DOES THE CREATOR HAVE STANDARDS FOR HIS CREATION?

The purpose of this work is to reveal what has been missing in our knowledge of the Creator's design for humanity. *Preparation for the End: Moral and Natural Law* reveals the cause of man's suffering; if we choose to follow God's standards man's suffering may be alleviated and ultimately eliminated. The intention is to illuminate the return path to the original sinless nature of our ancestors Adam and Eve before the fall. Once we choose to know and follow Jeshua's standards, His grace will make it possible to do so.

"...prepare ye the way of the people; cast up, cast up the highway; gather out the stones; lift up a standard for the people." Is. 62:10 Prophets don't always tell the future but they do call people to the truth.

Note: All biblical references in this work are from The King James Version of the Holy Bible which is both historically and mathematically accurate.

Christ said, "...I am come that they may have life and that they might have it more abundantly...I am the good shepherd; the good shepherd giveth his life for the sheep." John 10:10-11

"...thus saith the Lord: Behold I set before you the way of life, and the way of death." Jer. 21:8

For all of his scientific advancements man has not been able to create life from scratch.

It is moral to stand for life on all levels.

The Bible teaches that the life is in the blood. In addition, "...all things are cleansed with blood Gen. 9:4 "...without shedding of blood there is no forgiveness (of sin)." Heb. 9:22

Sin (error) brings suffering. The ultimate healing made possible by Christ's complete sacrifice encompasses the whole person, alleviating and eliminating the mental, emotional and physical sufferings that result from sin.

We can't know within ourselves our sinful condition. "The heart is deceitful above all things. and desperately wicked: who can know it?" Jer. 17:9 Humans rationalize behavior. Only God can show us our true state but that can't happen unless we surrender to Him and His leading. The Torah (the Law) and The Laws of Nature show the way.

Pride causes us to think we are fine and that we have arrived at all the truth. "...thou sayest I am rich, and increased with goods, and have need of nothing; ...knowest not that thou art wretched, and miserable, and poor, and blind and naked:" Rev. 3:17

"...strait is the gate, and narrow is the way, which leadeth unto life, and few be there that find it." Matt. 7:14 God's people will be learning for eternity!

"The spirit of the Lord God is upon me; because the Lord hath annointed me to preach good tidings unto the meek; he hath sent me to bind up the brokenhearted, to proclaim liberty to the captives, and the opening of the prison to them that are bound...to comfort all that mourn...to give them beauty for ashes, the oil of joy for mourning, the garment of praise for the spirit of heaviness; that they might be called trees of righteousness, the planting of the Lord, that he might be glorified. And they shall build up the old wastes, they shall raise up the former desolations, and they shall repair the waste cities; the desolations of many generations." Is. 61:1-4

"I have set watchmen on thy walls, O Jerusalem (God's people), which shall never hold their peace day nor night; ye that make mention of the Lord, keep not silence." Is. 62:6 Noah forewarned of a coming calamity and was called a fanatic. When the flood came it was too late for the people to be saved.

It's time to rebuild the streets (paths) and walls (laws) even in troublous times.

"And they that shall be of thee shall build the old waste places; thou shall raise up the foundations of many generations; and thou shalt be called, the repairer of the breach, the restorer of paths to dwell in." Is. 58:12

Thus saith the Lord, "Stand ye in the ways, and see, and ask for the old paths, where is the good way, and walk therein, and ye shall find rest for your souls." Jer. 6:16

"Now hearken, O Israel (now God's people), unto the statutes and unto the judgments, which I teach you, for to do them, that ye may live, and go in and possess the land which the LORD God of your fathers giveth you. Ye shall not add unto the word which I command you, neither shall ye diminish aught from it, that ye may keep the commandments of the LORD your God which I command you." Deut 4:1-2 God changeth not. His Word applies for all times which is reiterated in the New Testament, "And if any man shall take away from the words of this prophecy, God shall take away his part out of the book of life, and out of the holy city, and from the things which are written in this book, the book of life, and out of the holy city, and from the things which are written in this book." Rev. 22:19

The moral laws and the laws of our constitutional bodies are of equal import.

"The law of the Lord is perfect, converting the soul..." Ps. 19:7 According to Gen. 2:7 The soul is the combination of the dust of the ground infused with God's breath of life.

"...sin is transgression of the law." 1 John 3:4 "I had not known sin, but by the law." Rom. 7:7

The motivation behind evil is to eliminate the knowledge of and adherence to moral and natural law.

We live in a fallen world characterized by rebelliousness. Humanity fell on appetite (desire) which is the final test in these end times. We need to take the return path to the original intention of God who made man in His image. "Declaring the end from the beginning." Is. 46:10

Freedom is available once we are governed by God's laws both moral and natural.

Here are several key definitions to assist in our understanding:

Repentance is the result of conviction and is a change of mind. Humbling oneself to the Creator and His laws. "I acknowledge my sin unto thee and mine iniquity have I not hid. I said I will confess my transgressions unto the Lord; and thou forgavest the iniquity of my sin..." Ps. 32:5

Conversion is a change of character, values and conduct usually signified by a public baptism. Conversion is a voluntary exercise of the will. True conversion to Christianity is a personal, internal matter and can never be forced. This entails a whole new direction in life; from a lax to a more earnest and serious way of life which embraces God and rejects sin which includes a personal commitment to a life of holiness.

Revival is a renewal of spiritual life. A quickening of the powers of mind and heart – a return to primitive godliness.

Reformation is a reorganization in thinking, a change of ideas and theories, habits and practices.

Revival and reformation must blend in knowing and honoring moral and natural law.

The law points out sin and reveals the obedient life.

Grace removes sin and makes the obedient life a reality.

Now let's take a look at the impact following moral law can have on our lives.

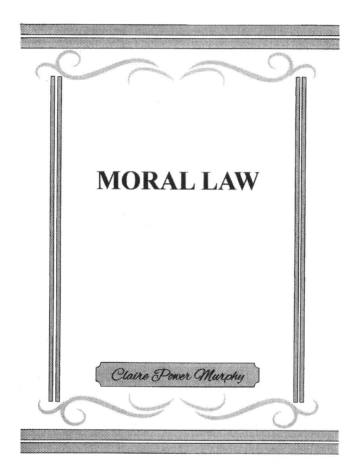

MORAL LAW

Claire Power Murphy

HAVE you heard the familiar cry, "...judgment is turned away backward, and justice standeth afar off: for truth is fallen in the street and equity cannot enter." Is. 59:14 We live in world of unreality steeped in fraud in banking, government, law, education, religion and health. Inspiring role models are few and far between. The hatred of Satan towards the followers of the true Christ is intensifying. Spiritualism, in the form of man's philosophies, pantheism, and the "love" gospel, has resulted in people not being in agreement, based on the Bible, as to what is right and what is wrong. Each has set up his own god and God's mishpat (law to judgment) has been all but destroyed. Scripture is clear that when mishpat is gone God acts to allow a people to reap the results of their rejection of His mishpat, and the people are destroyed by satanic power. Know that miracles do not produce faith. "Faith comes by hearing the word of God". Rom. 10:17 Take heart dear reader. We have the blessed assurance that Christ is far mightier than Satan and will protect His people who abide in the hollow of His hand.

"Think not that I am come to destroy the law, or the prophets: I am not come to destroy, but to fulfill." Matt. 5:17 The law of God is the very heart of the scriptures. The Torah (the first five books of the Old Testament) is the matrix of our freedom. The law defines sin which establishes the need for a Savior. We are not, nor can we, be saved in sin. When a person no longer needs to worry about sin, the law of God, or the warnings of conscience he is prepared for spiritualism. "Do we...make void the law through faith? God forbid: yea we establish the law." Rom. 3:21 "...by the law is the knowledge of sin." Rom. 3:20 "...all have sinned, and come short of the glory of God." Rom 3:23

How may real peace be attained? Genuine peace may be received only through the truth by which we are sanctified. Scripture interprets scripture. Human reason results in something other than the truth. Sola Scriptura stands above the interpretation of man's church. The Bible is not just a theory. It's a living experience: reproving, instructing and most importantly giving us hope! Truth never places her delicate feet in a path of uncleanness or impurity. She brings all up to a high exalted level (a higher standard). Truth never makes people course, rough, or discourteous. Under the influence of Christ's discipline they are sanctified through the truth. Truth is not about you but rather the Word of God.

Never base your faith on how you feel but rather on what God says.

Humanity is at a crossroads. Our spirituality and free will are under attack. One of God's conditional promises is most applicable, "And I will walk among you, and will be your God, and ye shall be my people. ...But if ye will not hearken unto me, and will not do all my commandments; And if ye shall despise my statutes, or if you should abhor my judgments...I also will do this unto you; I will ever appoint over you terror..." Lev. 26: 12-16 The statutes protect the ten commandments. The key to sanctification is keeping God's holy feasts wherein are explained the work of redemption. For more on this subject visit www.lightedway.org

The body of Christ is not a religion. There are thousands of denominations. The practice of religiosity is political. Belief in anything does not make it real. We must mourn for the sins committed in the church to receive the comfort of the Holy Spirit. Religion is not intended to be emotional but rather factual.

"...my people have forgotten me, they have burned incense to vanity, and they have caused them to stumble in their ways from the ancient paths...in a way not cast up." Jer. 19:15

Blinded by the Temple the Jews interpreted the scripture by human reason. When the Messiah came they knew him not. Only those who were free from the Jewish Mishnah, the Jewish hermeneutic and exegesis were able to recognize the Christ. It is essential to be God governed as opposed to man managed. Conscience is either submitted to the Word of God or the church. Leaders teach that virtue is better than vice, but God being removed, they place their dependence on human power which by itself is worthless. We are made perfect only through surrendering to God's absolute authority in the scriptures. The ship that is going through are those who obey Yahweh by manifesting His righteous character in thought and deed. Simply put the vast subject of righteousness is holiness, likeness to God. It is conformity to the law of God; "...for all thy commandments are righteous." Ps. 119:172 We receive righteousness not by gifts or sacrifices, but it is given freely to every soul who hungers and thirsts for it thus adding a divine element to the life.

Through faith the believer passes from the position of a rebel, a child of sin and Satan, to the position of a loyal subject of Christ Jesus, not because of an inherent goodness, but because Christ receives him as His child by adoption. The sinner receives the forgiveness of his sins because these sins are borne by his Substitute and Surety. Jesus speaks to his heavenly Father saying, "This is My child, I reprieve him from the condemnation of death, giving him My life insurance policy (eternal life) because I have taken his place and have suffered for his sins." Thus man is pardoned and clothed with the beautiful garments of Christ's righteousness. A saved man has a clear conscience and is not against God or man; with Yahweh it is impossible to have a sick mind. "For God hath not given us the spirit of fear but of power and of love, and of a sound mind." 2Tim. 1:7

Do you know why you were born? Do you have a goal? God says, "I know the thoughts that I think toward you...thoughts of peace and not of evil, to give you an expected end." Jer. 19:11

The goal is to be written in the Lamb's Book of Life to enjoy the expected end of eternity with Him.

Do you desire to be one of God's people? "For the Lord hath chosen Zion (a people devoted to God); he hath desired it for his habitation." Ps. 132:13 Realize that even though our profession of faith may proclaim the theory of religion, it is our practical piety that demonstrates the word of truth. "...as God hath said, I will dwell in them and walk in them; and I will be their God, and they shall be my people." II Cor. 6:16 a thought which segues into the next section of this book which deals with Natural Law.

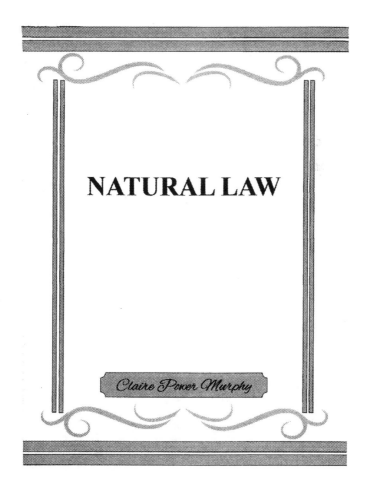

NATURAL LAW

Claire Power Murphy

PEOPLE are becoming progressively deceived and are walking after the imagination of their own hearts. "... Because they have forsaken my law which I set before them, and haven't obeyed my voice, neither walked therein...I will feed them...with wormwood and give them water of gall to drink." Jer. 9:13

Following Natural Law propels an individual to a higher frequency. Coupled with Moral Law one can rise above their circumstances.

Humanity has fallen into hypnotic seduction causing individuals to live for the moment. They are literally forfeiting their consciousness and subsequently their conscience. Further, humanity is being progressively enslaved physically, mentally, emotionally and spiritually descending into insensitivity and atheism thus causing a loss of moral and internal values.

And what was man's original condition? "And the Lord God formed man of the dust of the ground, and breathed into his nostrils the breath of life; and man became a living soul." Gen. 2:7 Man has unique human chromosomes which gives evidence that there is no basis for the theory of evolution. The genome is too complex to just happen as are the universes. We are left without excuse. Our Genetic Code is a set of rules defining how the four-letter code of DNA is translated into the 20-letter code of amino acids which are the building blocks of proteins essential for the growth and repair of animal tissue. The Genetic Code is a language of letters: A, T, C, and G proving that we were created from an intelligent mind. Sadly, man has lost the blueprint to his Genetic Code. Further, genetic manipulation is happening in redesigning DNA by changing the chromosomes which are the genetic material of organisms and the planet's genome. It is a deception to believe that humans may become as gods and be programmed to live longer. Gen. 3:3-5 tells us that Yahshua is the only way to live forever. In Ex. 4:11 the Lord tells us that he made us. Products function best when the directions for use are read and then followed. It is important to note that only humans created in God's image can be saved. The good news is that there are solutions in following His laws, praying without ceasing, and, in returning to man's original natural perfected condition.

There are many interpretations for The Mark of the Beast. In fact any deviation from the Creator's original design and plan will result in receiving the mark. The RFID (radio-frequency identification) chip has often been called the Mark. However, it is just a stepping stone. God's plan for man was a 2 strand DNA which included the miracle of life created by God and The Tree of Life to sustain it. However, when Adam and Eve partook of the Tree of Knowledge of Good and Evil they added a 3rd strand which now includes the Magic of Satan which may only be overcome through submitting to the Creator's laws for life. We are being prepared for the Mark through movies such as *Mark III*, *Iron Man, Man of Steel,* and *Born This Way.* Iron and clay are being mixed – computer with flesh (machine with man).

The number 666 relates to the carbon atom and man. Carbon-12, one of the 5 elements in the human DNA, is composed of 6 protons, 6 electron and 6 neutrons which is actually created in the stars; as Carl Sagan once said, "We're made of star stuff". Phosphous (Lucifer) is the 'spark' in our DNA that make us fire. When the 666 of carbon is combined with other elements and mixed with Phosp-Horus, we get a combination or reaction of chemical elements that forms DNA and RNA. This chemical carrier is the very code for all life. Various chemical elements, when combined with carbon, form our very material reality or what some may call the matrix. The Earth, and all who inhabit it, are becoming increasingly carbonized (darkened, polluted) and are now at the very tippy-toes of the image in Daniel. It is the design of Satan to seek to addict and restrict us to the dense physical senses. Indeed, one interpretation of the Number of the Beast (666) is that Antichrist is the number of a man. It is at this level the individual needs to reform. As one climbs the ladder of health he becomes freer from gravity and the forces which cause man to stay connected with the Earth and subsequently comes into in a better position to catch a glimpse of heaven.

In a sea of pollution man is increasingly dealing with nanoparticles (foreign substances) in the air, water, soil and subsequently food. It is the common belief that these contaminated substances remain in the body causing bio accumulation, sickness and ultimately death. Such need not be the case. There are definitely ways to eliminate toxins through cleansing, fasting and upgrading. For answers see the author's book, *The 8 Laws of Health with Recipes.*

Another problem which now confronts humanity is the increase in radiation on the planet particularly in the Northern Hemisphere. All life is being affected especially that in the Pacific Ocean which is referred to in the last book of the Bible, Revelation, as one third of the seas. As a result there is a crack in the food chain beginning with radiated plankton contaminating any food from the sea and resulting in a key source of oxygen being depleted as well. There is an increase in thyroid cancer and also problems with newborns. The intention of the enemy is to eliminate all of God's image on the planet. Iodine is most definitely recommended, but, just one antidote is hardly sufficient to counteract the huge onslaught. A lifestyle change is most definitely in order.

Further, neutron bombardment is crystallizing metal structures; for example more planes are falling apart. Pilots, flight attendants and frequent fliers who spend much time in the highly radioactive air column at 30,000 feet are becoming sick. The Chernobyl Disaster and the Fukushima Daichi Disaster are among the main causes of global hypothyroidism and graves disease to the present and future generations. We are experiencing ongoing attacks on Iodine and Earth's Magnetic

Shield. An organic vegan diet free from fluoride, aspartame, aminosweet, MSG, gluten, sugars, and other toxins is necessary leading to the ultimate nutrition which is fruit, grains and nuts. The pH of Earth and all living things must be alkalized over 7 for progressive survival!

Inbreeding of various bloodlines through genetic procreation has resulted in deficiencies in their blood causing energetic information to shift within the decoding system of the brain. Over generations the reptilian portion of the brain has become stronger requiring greater focus to maintain its human shape. It feeds well on human blood, particularly that of the young, and, often attempts to seek gratification through pedaphilia. All that it is seeking is the minerals which its own blood so desperately craves, especially iron. It need not take blood (iron, energy) from another. It needs to take the blood (juice) from the natural produce of the earth to heal itself. This shapeshifting is alterable with proper fueling of the organism. Then he will be satisfied in a natural environment and will seek to preserve what remains and will long to spend eternity with Jesus in the New Earth when all will be restored to even better than the original design. The path is a return to the original Rx for humanity.

Traditional/allopathic medicine is currently being challenged by alternative/complementary medicine which is more natural than the traditional but still offers solutions to specific problems. Only altering the fuel (food) of the organism will produce a whole and complete upgrade.

There is an increasing manifestation of evil spirits on the planet. Know that most occurrences are the result of diseased conditions which open the door to possession. Emerging diseases (lack of ease) are resulting from the increase of neuro toxins and drugs most recently flakka.

There is great concern about vaccines and their potential harmful effects both in the physical and in the psyche. Rather than being fearful recognize that the combination of faith in God coupled with the effects of a high level lifestyle may counteract the counterfeit.

Contemplating God will change your brain. The more we know about Him the more we come to love Him and want to please and obey Him. Beginning each morning with prayer leads to new brain cells being created every day. New baby dendrites (the branched parts of nerve cells) lead to a sanctified life. "They are new every morning..." Lam. 3:23

In Gen. 2:16 we learn that temperance was the first great moral lesson which was to check man's appetite (desires). God had given man in his perfect state the fruits of the earth for food. When man lost Eden he was banned from the battery charger, The Tree of Life. Knowing man would degenerate, God mercifully gave him the idea of extracting the juice of plant life in order to gain its finest nourishment. Now man also has the capacity to juice mega doses of life enabling him to imbibe life-giving minerals and enzymes for his health. Following man's fall God mercifully gave man the herb of the field to consume; the vegetation being required for the healing of the body especially in the megadoses yielded through juicing.

Sadly man rejected the admonition not to consume of the Tree of Knowledge of Good and Evil which has caused mankind to deteriorate and consume increasingly from The Tree of Death leading into the dark last days.

Since Lucifer fell and was banished from heaven to the Earth he became known as Satan and was granted dominion over the earth. As such he and his imps (other fallen angels) have worked tirelessly to exert their influence over mankind. A corrupted seed was found in Adam and Eve's murderous son Cain and has been passed down through the generations. When fallen angels mixed with human women the seed became manifested in bloodlines thirsty for power. Man will never be fully satisfied without submitting to the Lord and His ways which includes a balanced blood chemistry replete with all of the basic twelve minerals which were in the original soil from which man was created.

As in the days of Noah man is not in God's image. Man is eating and drinking the wrong things. He needs to be en route back to the original in all ways. Noah and his family were preserved. In Gen. 6:9 we learn that Noah was perfect in his geneology. And what do you think will preserve man once again?

For thousands of years man knew there would be a Savior. Even before the scriptures at the fall God rearranged the stars into pictograms known as constellations to tell the story of redemption.

In preparation for a coming Savior man offered bloody sacrifices of untold innocent lambs. Christ did come right on time and fulfilled the prophecies and the law. The blessed hope was realized that man would henceforth have the opportunity to be born again which applies to the physical as well. While it is true that we inherit 'the original sin' from our ancestors both spiritually and physically, the good news is that in both cases the sin may not only be overcome but that we may also grow in grace, strength and resilience. While the body is being cleansed and the accumulated dross of generations of sin is being removed, the process upsets the flesh. The good news is that with a strengthened immune system the devil can no longer dictate to you by ruling your flesh!

Cleanse the soul temple of its defilement that Christ may come in and reign supreme. Laminin, whose function is to hold everything together, is in the form of a cross and lives lives in every cell of our body. The idea is to clear it of foreign matter so Christ may express more freely through us. The key to a healthy life lies in a whole uninterrupted circulation of life-giving balanced blood. Multi award-winning

Preserved to Serve offers irrefutable proof in support of this declaration!

Appetite (intemperance) is the base temptation to all others. Like Esau man has sold his birthright (salvation) for food. "Know ye not that ye are the temple of God, and that the spirit of God dwelleth in you? If any man defile the temple of God, him shall God destroy; for the temple of God is holy, which temple ye are." 1Cor. 3:16-17 With all that has been said about how we should treat our bodies, appetite is the great law which governs humanity. Overcoming appetite gives moral power to overcome all other temptations leaving nothing in us to respond to Satan. First man must see the need for temperance which includes his desires. He needs to ask for moderation since it is a gift from the Holy Spirit. Finally, man must receive it and act upon it with God's help. It is through faith that man overcomes battles with self; the last great one being the battle of the appetite. "Behold, I stand at the door, and knock, if any man hears my voice, and opens the door I will come into him, and will sup with him, and he with me." Rev. 3:20

Man was created in God's image. He had a perfect body, diet and character. Adam and Eve fell on appetite. Moses fasted prior to receiving the law (The Torah). Elijah fasted prior to upholding the law. John the Baptist lived simply prior to introducing the coming of the Savior who was to fulfill the law. Christ (in the flesh) was tempted sorely when weak and hungered at the end of a forty day fast. He maintained a close connection to the Father throughout and would not yield to Satan's offer of the whole Earth if Christ would just worship Him. If these men overcame 'in the flesh' so can we with God's help. Jeshua promises to give strength to the feint. We are admonished not to eat for drunkenness if we are to return to our original intended state.

The richest possession man can have is health without which happiness is an illusion.

Overcoming appetite is the key.

Why live healthfully?

- For good physical health with a minimum of medical bills
- We are not our own by creation and redemption

- Be holy as God is holy
- Serve God with all our might, mind and strength
- Possess a clear mind capable of discerning truth
- "Do all to the glory of God." 1Cor. 10:31

A common belief is that the universal language of music influences our behavior. While partially true it is the level of harmony and balance within the individual which gravitates towards certain types of music. The brain waves need to be balanced in order to receive harmonious God-like impulses which cause the spirit to grow and flourish. Old hymns contain this type of music, rhythm and messages of truth which cause the frontal lobes (the spiritual portion of the brain) to be activated. On the other hand drumming, and emphasis on a beat, is straight out of voodoo and is causing many to be lost.

We are in need of a standard against which to measure true progress; that standard has been fully proven to be the chemistry of the life-giving blood and the balance of its mineral content; a fact irrefutably proven in the first book of "The Restoration Trilogy", multi award-winning

Preserved to Serve. It is here where the human agent can help himself to better health. The blood affects all parts of the body including the frontal lobes. Once the immune system is strengthened all else is much easier to achieve.

Many people are busy prepping for hard times. The greatest preparation is in our own temples. The higher the quality of nutrition, the less food needs to be gathered. Daniel had the strength to stand for truth because he had the fortification of a simple diet without the King's meat and delicacies. Any true Christian planning on standing for the truths found in the Bible had best pay attention to boosting his/her health as a strong support system during this key preparation period.

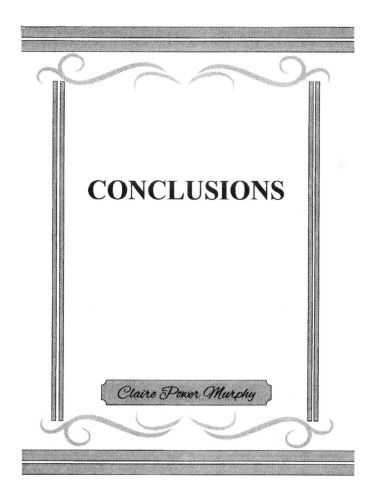

CONCLUSIONS

Claire Power Murphy

"THE LAW of the Lord is perfect, converting the soul; the testimony of the Lord is sure, making wise the simple." Ps. 19:7 *Preparation for the End: Moral and Natural Law* has demonstrated the connection between one's moral and natural condition. We are admonished to "...glorify God in your body, and in your spirit which are God's." 1Cor 6:20 We live in a temple of fallen nature. Yah's people are the sanctuary. In order to improve and ascend to higher spiritual levels, they are to be sober and clear minded and not impaired by faulty nutrition and ultimately drugs which affect the Most Holy Place which is the mind.

Paul, the most prolific contributor to the New Testament, wrote clearly on this subject, "...I keep under my body, and bring it into subjection: lest that, by any means, when I have preached to others, I myself should be a castaway." 1Cor. 9:27 He further exhorts, "I beseech you therefore, brethren, by the mercies of God, that ye present your bodies a living sacrifice, holy, acceptable unto God, which is your reasonable service. And be not conformed to this world: be ye transformed by the renewing of your mind..." Rom. 12:1-2

Claire Power Murphy

Contemplating God will change your mind. We are to be praying constantly, especially in the morning when God may refresh us by growing new baby dendrites leading to a sanctified life. "They are new every morning..." Lam. 3:23 We are to pray for everyone, ourselves, families, friends and even our enemies. We must let go of sin or we will be destroyed with it. Whether therefore ye eat, or drink, or whatever ye do. Do all to the glory of God." 1Cor. 10:31

It is the writer's prayer that stony hearts will become fleshy through surrendering their whole being to Jesus and His merciful laws. It's not about our 'rights'. Freedom occurs when we are no longer mad at God and become at peace. Fear is a form of idolatry, worshipping that which you fear. Through getting to know Him fear is transmuted to trust in Yah wherein lies perfect peace when following His law.

It is time to be prepping to become one of the 144,000 who walk in the path of righteousness. We need to be growing in grace and holiness right now. Holiness is the finish line for the sanctified life. "Be ye therefore perfect even as your Father which is in heaven is perfect." Matt. 5:45 We need to be en route to becoming more like our Savior bearing His image, imitating His example and living His life. The process involves eliminating spiritual and physical bondage. "...let us cleanse ourselves from all filthiness of the flesh and spirit, perfecting holiness in the fear of God." II Cor. 7:1 Heaven may be attained by every one of us if we will strive do the will of Jesus and subsequently grow into His image. Humanity will regain the kingdom on appetite.

"...Blessed is he that watcheth, and keepeth his garments (white robes of righteousness), lest he walk naked, and they see his shame." Rev. 1:15 We receive His imputed righteousness at baptism but become fit (sanctified) by the imparting of His righteousness when we keep all of His holy days as a dress rehearsal in preparation for doing so for all eternity. Simultaneously, we need to be returning to a fruit diet which was the original diet and will be the diet for all eternity. Rev. 22:2 assures God's people that they will once again have access to the Tree of Life which bears twelve manner of fruits. There must be a union of the divine with the human for entrance into the Holy City. The Bible wraps around from the beginning to the end to the beginning again. It's time to return to the original plan for humanity before the fall. For more on this subject the author recommends reading the second book in the "Restoration Trilogy", *Towards the 144,000*.

"I have set before you life and death, blessing and cursing: therefore choose life, that both thou and thy seed may live." Deut. 30:19 When Jeshua returns we will either reflect His glory or be consumed by it.

Once new light is shone we have a responsibility to move towards following it. The quality of nutrition affects the personality which also affects the character. The higher the quality of nutrition ingested the greater the spiritual understanding and ability to follow it.

Christ is returning for His righteous people who will be manifesting the fruit of the spirit, "...love, joy, peace, meekness, temperance..." Gal. 5: 22-23

God changes not. His laws are eternal!

Printed in the United States
By Bookmasters